Monograph on
Dizziness

Monograph on Dizziness

Editors

V Natarajan MD DM(Neurology)
FRCP(Edinburgh) FAAN FIAN FIMSA
Former Professor and Head
Madras Institute of Neurology
Madras Medical College
Professor Emeritus
The Tamil Nadu Dr MGR Medical University
Chennai, Tamil Nadu, India

K Mugundhan MD DM(Neurology)
FRCP(Edinburgh, London, Glasgow, Ireland)
FACP FICP FIMSA
Professor and Head
Department of Neurology
Stanley Medical College
Chennai, Tamil Nadu, India

Forewords
Jyotirmoy Pal
Girish Mathur

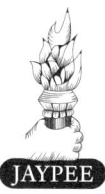

JAYPEE BROTHERS MEDICAL PUBLISHERS
The Health Sciences Publisher
New Delhi | London

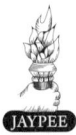 **Jaypee Brothers Medical Publishers (P) Ltd**

Headquarters
EMCA House
23/23-B, Ansari Road, Daryaganj
New Delhi 110 002, India
Landline: +91-11-23272143, +91-11-23272703
+91-11-23282021, +91-11-23245672
E-mail: jaypee@jaypeebrothers.com

Corporate Office
Jaypee Brothers Medical Publishers (P) Ltd.
4838/24, Ansari Road, Daryaganj
New Delhi 110 002, India
Phone: +91-11-43574357
Fax: +91-11-43574314
E-mail: jaypee@jaypeebrothers.com

Overseas Office
JP Medical Ltd.
83, Victoria Street, London
SW1H 0HW (UK)
Phone: +44-20 3170 8910
Fax: +44(0)20 3008 6180
E-mail: info@jpmedpub.com

Website: www.jaypeebrothers.com
Website: www.jaypeedigital.com

© 2024, Jaypee Brothers Medical Publishers

The views and opinions expressed in this book are solely those of the original contributor(s)/author(s) and do not necessarily represent those of editor(s) or publisher of the book.

All rights reserved. No part of this publication may be reproduced, stored or transmitted in any form or by any means, electronic, mechanical, photocopying, recording or otherwise, without the prior permission in writing of the publishers.

All brand names and product names used in this book are trade names, service marks, trademarks or registered trademarks of their respective owners. The publisher is not associated with any product or vendor mentioned in this book.

Medical knowledge and practice change constantly. This book is designed to provide accurate, authoritative information about the subject matter in question. However, readers are advised to check the most current information available on procedures included and check information from the manufacturer of each product to be administered, to verify the recommended dose, formula, method and duration of administration, adverse effects and contraindications. It is the responsibility of the practitioner to take all appropriate safety precautions. Neither the publisher nor the author(s)/editor(s) assume any liability for any injury and/or damage to persons or property arising from or related to use of material in this book.

This book is sold on the understanding that the publisher is not engaged in providing professional medical services. If such advice or services are required, the services of a competent medical professional should be sought.

Every effort has been made where necessary to contact holders of copyright to obtain permission to reproduce copyright material. If any have been inadvertently overlooked, the publisher will be pleased to make the necessary arrangements at the first opportunity.

Inquiries for bulk sales may be solicited at: jaypee@jaypeebrothers.com

Monograph on Dizziness / V Natarajan, K Mugundhan

First Edition: **2024**

ISBN: 978-93-5696-510-2

Printed at: Sterling Graphics Pvt. Ltd. India

Foreword

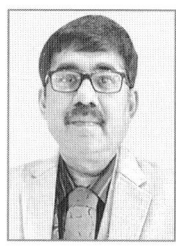

Jyotirmoy Pal MD FRCP(London, Glasgow, Edinburgh)
FICP FACP WHO Fellow
Dean, Indian College of Physicians

It gives me immense pleasure to present the *"Monograph on Dizziness"* with an aim to provide a practical approach to differential diagnosis and clinical analysis of this common presentation.

This book will be of immense help in day-to-day practice of our colleagues and a ready reckoner for the practitioners for decision-making and investigation.

I once again congratulate Dr V Natarajan and Dr K Mugundhan for this wonderful effort and wish them all the best for the success of this publication.

Foreword

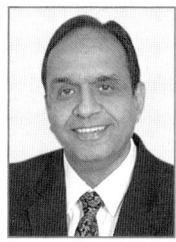

Girish Mathur MD FICP FACP FRCP(London, Glasgow, Edinburgh)
FIACM FRSSDI Fellow Diabetes India
President, Association of Physicians of India

In the complex realm of human health, there are conditions that often defy easy understanding and leave those affected searching for answers. Dizziness, seemingly innocuous in its name, is one such condition that can profoundly disrupt the lives of those who experience it.

In this innovative "*Monograph on Dizziness*", Dr K Mugundhan and Dr V Natarajan delve deep into the intricate realm of dizziness. Their meticulous research and expertise in the field shine through as they unravel the complexities of this common yet often misunderstood sensation. This comprehensive work promises to not only expand our understanding of dizziness but also pave the way for innovative approaches to diagnosis and treatment.

Dr Mugundhan and Dr Natarajan bring to this book a wealth of knowledge and a dedication to unraveling the mysteries of dizziness.

I believe that this monograph will prove to be a valuable resource for practicing physicians and postgraduate students in understanding the complex problem of dizziness.

Preface

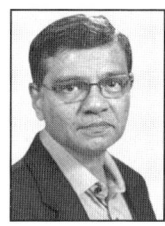

V Natarajan MD DM(Neurology)
FRCP(Edinburgh) FAAN FIAN FIMSA

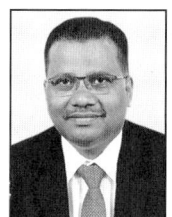

K Mugundhan MD DM(Neurology)
FRCP(Edinburgh, London, Glasgow, Ireland) FACP FICP FIMSA

Dizziness is a frequent and challenging symptom which the practitioner faces. It is frequently equated with vertigo though dizziness includes non vertiginous conditions and is hence challenging.

Obtaining a proper description of the symptom is essential but is difficult, as the patient invariably gives a vague and imprecise description needing probing and leading questions to elicit a meaningful description of the symptom.

"There can be few physicians so dedicated to their art that they do not experience a slight decline in spirits on learning that their patient's complaint is dizziness".
—In the words of Professor WB Matthew

The bedside evaluation of the dizzy patient is also formidable as multiple systems are involved.

Skill is required in examining the inner ear, brainstem, and the cerebellum and to interpret the findings.

This monograph is a concise, simplified narrative which would help the physician confidently manage the patient with dizziness.

A knowledgeable physician should be able to diagnose the cause of dizziness in more than 80% of patients and manage without recourse to extensive and expensive investigations by eliciting a good history and clinical examination.

This monograph is not exhaustive and does not purport to be a textbook covering all aspects but nevertheless should be an useful guide towards efficient management of the dizzy patient.

Acknowledgments

We are extremely grateful to Dr Jyotirmoy Pal and Dr Girish Mathur for their kind words in the foreword.

We are deeply indebted to our teachers Professors K Jagannathan, G Arjundas, K Srinivas, Zaheer Ahmed Sayeed, and CU Velmurugendran, all former professors at the Institute of Neurology, Chennai, whose inspiration and guidance have been the biggest strength and source of knowledge to the first author.

We are grateful to our colleagues Drs PR Sowmini, M Sathish Kumar, Assistant Professors of Neurology, Stanley Medical College, Chennai, Tamil Nadu, India, and Dr Ganesh V, Consultant Neurologist, Sri Lakshmi Narayana Institute of Medical Sciences, Puducherry, India, for their contribution with suggestions and help in corrections.

We would like to thank all our patients who were the true sources of the material for this book.

We would also like to extend our gratitude to our family members for their patience and support.

Thanks are due to the publishers for encouraging and putting up with us with repeated corrections.

We especially appreciate the constant support and encouragement of Shri Jitendar P Vij (Group Chairman) and Mr Ankit Vij (Managing Director) of M/s Jaypee Brothers Medical Publishers (P) Ltd., New Delhi, India, in publishing the book and also their associates, particularly Ms Chetna Malhotra (Senior Director—Professional Publishing, Marketing, and Business Development), and Ms Charu Lata (Development Editor), who have been prompt, efficient, and most helpful.

Contents

PART 1: CLINICAL APPROACH TO DIZZINESS

Introduction	1
Symptom Analysis of the Types of Dizziness	2
Further History	3
Examination	6
Investigations	13
Differential Diagnosis of Vertigo	16

PART 2: DISORDERS CAUSING DIZZINESS

Disorders Causing Episodic Vestibular Syndrome	17
Benign Paroxysmal Positional Vertigo (BPPV)	17
Migrainous Vertigo or Vestibular Migraine	18
Ménière's Disease	22
Acute Vestibular Syndrome	24
Vestibular Neuritis/Vestibular Neuronitis	25
Labyrinthitis	26
Mal De Débarquement Syndrome (MdDS)	28
Superior Semicircular Canal Dehiscence	29
Chronic Vestibular Syndrome	30
Vestibular Paroxysmia	32
Vestibulogenic Seizure or Epileptic Vertigo	33
Drug-related Dizziness	34
Orthostatic Dizziness and other Causes of Dizziness	35
Postural Orthostatic Tachycardia Syndrome	35
Index	39

PART 1

Clinical Approach to Dizziness

■ INTRODUCTION

Dizziness and giddiness are used interchangeably by patients and refer to several descriptive symptoms collectively included under the above terms, and these descriptions make them difficult to understand.

These symptoms include:
- A sensation of spinning, either of the surroundings or of the self, with spinning of the head; and this symptom is referred to as vertigo, occurring due to vestibular system involvement.
- The other common description is a feeling of being pushed, and less often, of tilting or levitating, which also indicates dysfunction of the vestibular system.
- Another common description is that of feeling unsteady while walking, turning, or standing due to impairment of balance—a state of disequilibrium.
- A sensation of dimming of vision, a sinking feel, or a feeling of going to pass out are other descriptions indicating a state of presyncope or syncope per se.

The term 'giddy' or 'dizzy' expressed by the patient could mean any of the above symptoms and may also include a state of generalized weakness and anxiety. Hence, it becomes imperative to elicit from the patient directly, a detailed, and as accurate a history as possible. The attendant, even if it happens to be the wife or offspring, would not know what the patient experiences or has experienced. It would be pointless to elicit a history from them, even if the patient is unable to give a good description. This is the case quite often, making it difficult for the physician to understand the symptom. It is not easy for the patients to describe the details the way we want, and quite often, the description also keeps changing as more and more questions are asked of them. To complicate matters further, the relatives would chip in with their own understanding of the patient's symptoms, to confuse further.

SYMPTOM ANALYSIS OF THE TYPES OF DIZZINESS

Vertigo

This is a specific type of giddiness or dizziness in which the patient experiences the outside world to be spinning which is referred to as objective vertigo or the patient's head spinning inside which is referred to as subjective vertigo. Vertigo is not a separate disease process but, is a multisensory and sensorimotor syndrome with various etiologies and pathogenesis and has a lifetime prevalence of 20–30%.

The symptom could be worsened by movement of the head or neck, such as when looking up or down, turning to one side, rolling over, or getting into or out of bed. The patient could also experience a feeling of being tilted or pushed, and at times, being pushed backwards. This symptom is an indication of dysfunction of the vestibular system about which we shall discuss later. Vertigo is a symptom and not a diagnostic entity, though many patients and even doctors believe it to be so. It is not uncommon to see patients being treated continuously for months and even years as vertigo, for symptoms of dizziness with betahistines and calcium channel blockers, wherein they were not necessary. This happens as the symptom, vertigo is misunderstood and used erroneously to designate symptoms described below, leading to irrelevant investigations and possibly inappropriate treatment.

Imbalance

Imbalance or a state of disequilibrium is quite often referred to by patients as 'giddiness' when they have a sense of losing balance on standing or walking, or a feeling that they might fall while walking or turning, especially on uneven ground or in the dark, without having spinning or a sense of rotation. It is an indication of a disorder of gait, and evaluation for neurological disorders that cause gait dysfunction has to be carried out.

Presyncope

A cardiovascular disorder or massive blood loss can cause low blood pressure or reduced blood flow to the brain which results in the patient experiencing a dimming of the vision associated with the feeling of sinking or losing consciousness, along with palpitations or sweating. This might occur when the patient stands up or is in an upright position, and after exertion, or pressure over the neck by tight clothing, and is aggravated by rotating the neck, causing vagotonia. Such an experience is also described as giddiness by the patient, and in such situations, blood pressure needs to be checked in lying and standing positions at least on three occasions to exclude postural hypotension. This patient also needs to be evaluated for an underlying cardiac disorder.

Lightheadedness

Other descriptions given by patients as 'giddiness' would include lightheadedness or a heavy feel of the head, apart from tingling or numbness in the head associated with an inability to think or concentrate, and a wobbly feel within the head. These symptoms are often due to stress, depression, or feelings of insecurity. At times, these could indicate milder versions of the symptom complexes described earlier and one would have to enquire regarding occurrence of the triggers of the previously described conditions, to see whether it would fit into one of those conditions.

▌FURTHER HISTORY

After analyzing the type of dizziness and obtaining a detailed description of the symptom experienced by the patient, other details regarding the medications being currently taken and exposure to toxins have to be enquired. Dizziness can occur as an adverse effect of a number of medications and a review of the medications, and their adverse effects would be of great value. These medications would include antiseizure medications (ASMs), antidepressants, antipsychotics, aminoglycosides, antiarrhythmogenic agents, antihypertensives, and antihistamines. A history of psychiatric, neurologic, cardiac, renal, hepatic illness, and comorbid disorders such as diabetes mellitus, dyslipidemia, hypertension, and hypothyroidism have to be ascertained.

After triaging the patient's symptoms based on the above details, the focus shifts to the evaluation of vertigo, which is the most common type of dizziness.

The four *T*s approach to vertigo would be helpful to remember, in which the four *T*s are:
1. *T*ypes of dizziness as outlined earlier and 'TiTrATE' where
2. *T*i – stands for timing,
3. *T*r – indicates the triggers, and
4. A*T*E – stands for targeted examination, and this provides an ideal format for the evaluation

Timing would include the onset, duration, and evolution of the attacks and whether they last for:
- Seconds to minutes;
- Minutes to hours; or
- Days

Triggers refer to positions of the body and head, head movements, actions like standing, walking, turning, or situational occurrence such as orthostatic posture, Valsalva maneuver, or sound exposure. It could also occur spontaneously without any trigger.

A history of the features associated with the giddiness, helps in pointing to the diagnosis and these features include:
- Unilateral ear fullness, muffled hearing, a roaring tinnitus preceding or in association with the giddiness, all of which would indicates the possibility of Ménière's disease (MD).

- Sensory, motor, or visual disturbances which are accompaniments of transient ischemic attacks (TIAs).
- Associated ataxia, dysarthria, and visual disturbances that signify a cerebellar cause.
- Abnormal hearing of internal body sounds (autophony) which is a feature of superior canal dehiscence.
- Anxiety that can be an underlying cause or could occur as a reaction to the accompanying apprehension.

Vertigo is due to a disorder of the vestibular system, which comprises the vestibular end organs, vestibular division of the eighth nerve, vestibular nuclei in the brainstem, and their connections to the cerebellum.

The vestibular system could be considered to be the sixth sense organ, apart from the eyes, nose, ears, tongue, and skin. It is an invisible system that takes part in posture control, gaze stabilization, orientation, perception of motion of self, memory in space of different locations, spatial relations between objects, and the integration of multiple sensations **(Figs. 1 and 2)**.

Based on the history, the occurrence of vertigo can be categorized into the following syndromes, and accordingly, their causes.

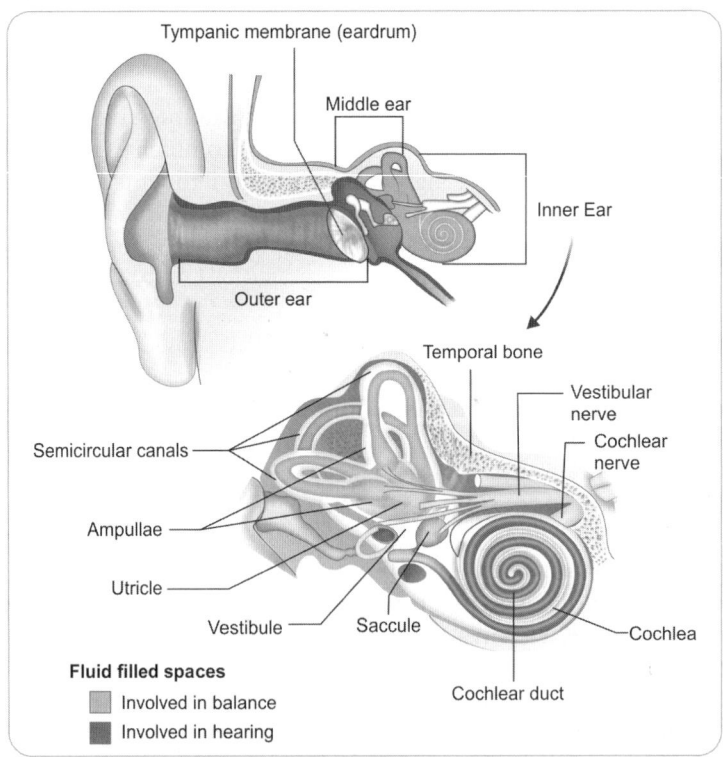

FIG. 1: Anatomy of the vestibular system includes three semicircular canals, utricle, and saccule.

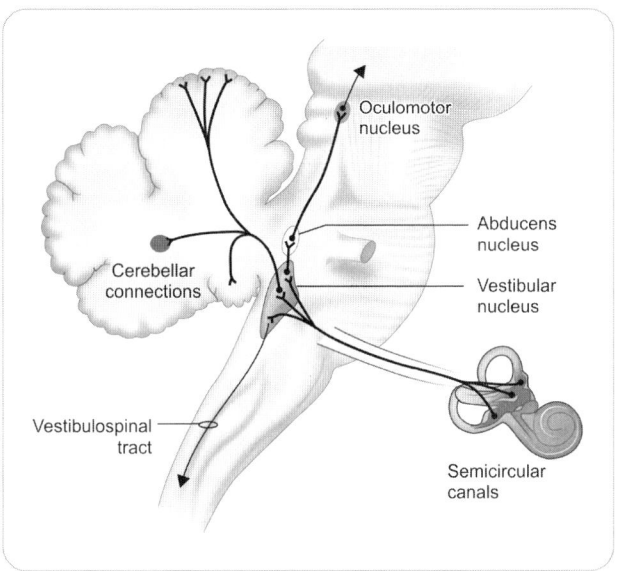

FIG. 2: Vestibular nuclei and their connections.

Episodic vestibular syndrome (EVS): It is characterized by intermittent, multiple, discrete episodes lasting for—
- Seconds to minutes—as in benign paroxysmal positional vertigo (BPPV) and vestibular paroxysmia
- Minutes to hours—in vestibular migraine, posterior circulation TIA, Ménière's disease, episodic ataxia type 2, and perilymphatic fistula
- Days—with vestibular migraine and multiple sclerosis

Acute vestibular syndrome (AVS): With acute onset and persistent dizziness lasting from days to weeks. It has a monophasic course, peaking of symptoms within a few days, and with fairly rapid improvement in a week, followed by more gradual improvement over weeks to months.

Acute vestibular syndrome can occur as a result of trauma, toxic exposure, or can be spontaneous.
- The traumatic syndrome occurs following blunt head trauma or blast injuries, which results in injury to the vestibular nerve, or concussion of the labyrinth, or disruption of inner ear membranes.
- Intoxication with ASMs, aminoglycosides, and carbon monoxide poisoning can cause a similar syndrome with dizziness, headaches, fatigue, unsteadiness of gait, and visual disturbances.
- The spontaneous AVS is characterized by an acute onset of continuous dizziness with vomiting, nystagmus, imbalance of gait, and inability to tolerate head movement, which lasts for days to weeks.

Patients are dizzy at rest, which gets aggravated with head movements. Conditions that cause spontaneous AVS include vestibular neuritis, posterior circulation strokes, Wernicke's encephalopathy, brainstem encephalitis, and demyelinating disease.

Chronic vestibular syndrome (CVS): It is characterized by persistent dizziness which lasts for weeks to months, and is associated with unsteadiness on walking, hearing impairment, and nystagmus and occurs with uncompensated unilateral vestibular loss, or cerebellar degeneration, or persistent perceptive postural dizziness.

▍EXAMINATION

Examination of a patient with vertigo should comprise of general examination, examination of the ear, and targeted examination of the vestibular neurologic systems.

The general examination should includes examination of the pulse for arrhythmias, blood pressure for changes in pressure in different postures, for anemia, for features of hypothyroidism, and the cardiovascular system evaluation for low output states, all of which could cause dizziness.

Examination of the ears should be done to look at the auricle, canal, and tympanic membrane. This should include the test for Hennebert's sign by pressing on the tragus and the external auditory meatus on the affected side to induce vertigo or nystagmus. Hearing impairment can be assessed by rubbing the fingers close to the ear and using the tuning fork of 256 Hz frequency for the Weber and Rinne tests for further evaluation if hearing is impaired.

The targeted examination of the vestibular system comprises of the—
- Head impulse test (HIT) or head thrust test (HTT) **(Figs. 3A and B)**
- Evaluation of nystagmus
- Test for skew

This battery of three tests is given the acronym of HINTS (Head Impulse, Nystagmus, Test for Skew) and has high reliability in the assessment of AVS with a sensitivity of 100% and specificity of 96% in ruling out stroke.

The Head Impulse Test

This maneuver tests the integrity of the vestibulo-ocular reflex and distinguishes brainstem and cerebellar strokes from peripheral acute vestibular disorders presenting with vertigo.

The test is performed by making the patient sit in front of the examiner and holding the patient's head steady in the midline. The patient is asked to fix his vision on the examiner's nose. Quick thrusts of the head are done rapidly without informing beforehand, with horizontal movements about 20° to either side, left and right, one after the other, and the saccadic movements of the eyes are observed. Normally, the eyes move in a direction opposite to that of the head movement. After the head movement is stopped, the patient's eye is observed on the side to which the head is turned for refixation saccade. The eyes should remain focused on the examiner's nose

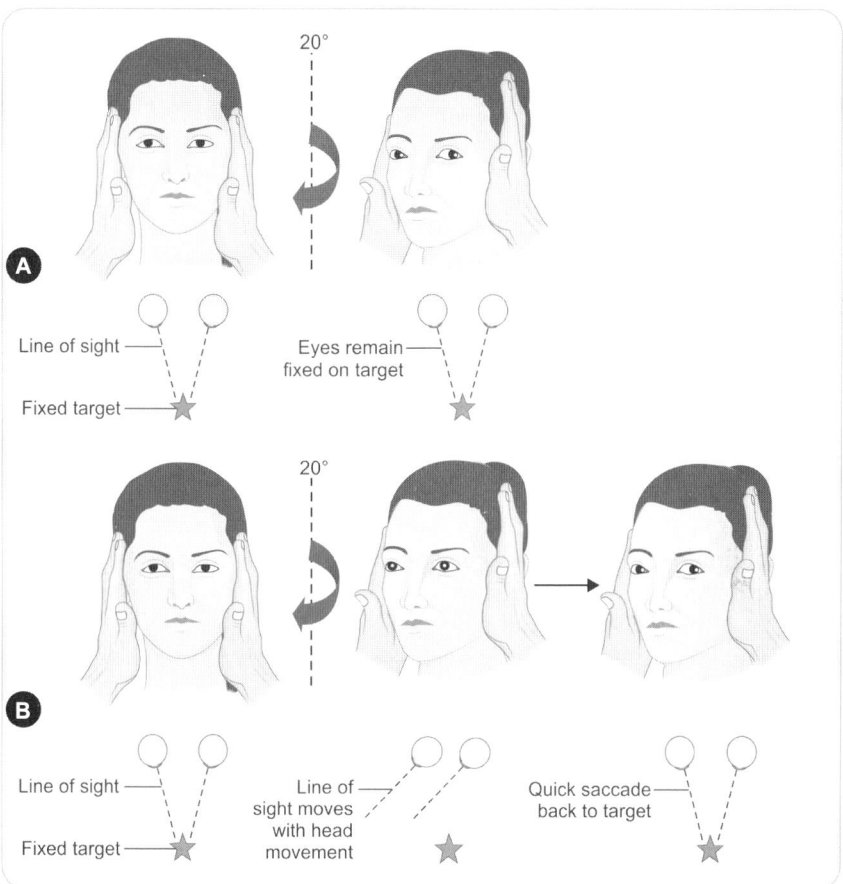

FIGS. 3A AND B: (A) The right ear has an intact peripheral vestibular function. When the head is turned to the right, the vestibulo-ocular reflex moves the eyes to maintain visual fixation. (B) The right ear now has impaired vestibular function. When the head is turned to the right, the eyes move with it, breaking visual fixation, and a refixation saccade is seen as the eyes dart back to the examiner's face. This indicates a peripheral vestibular disorder on the right side.

if the vestibulo-ocular reflex is intact when the test is considered negative. The test is abnormal or considered positive, if a corrective saccade is seen toward the affective side, to refixate on the examiner's nose.

The vestibulo-ocular reflex normally stabilizes the images on the fovea during head movements to provide clear vision. When the head moves, the vestibulo-ocular reflex is responsible for the eye movement, which is equal in magnitude to the head movement but in the opposite direction. However, in vestibulopathies, the eyes fail to correct for the head movement. The eyes move with the head and at the end of the head movement, the compensatory saccade corrects the error of gaze.

In patients with unilateral vestibulopathy, the corrective saccade occurs when the head is turned quickly toward the abnormal side. Left-sided saccades following a head thrust to the right would indicate right side abnormality, whereas right-sided saccades following left head thrust would indicate a left-sided vestibular pathology. If a normal response is elicited in a person with acute vertigo, it would indicate a central lesion as the cause of the vertigo.

Nystagmus

Nystagmus is an abnormal alternating slow and fast movement of the eyes and can be horizontal, vertical, or torsional. The main objective of evaluating nystagmus in a person with vertigo is to find out the site of pathology, whether it is in the brain or outside, i.e., a central lesion or a peripheral lesion.

A person with vertigo could show three types of nystagmus:
1. Spontaneous nystagmus (seen in primary position)
2. Gaze-evoked nystagmus (in eccentric eye positions), i.e., in the direction of gaze
3. Positional and positioning nystagmus (seen with change of head positions)

In acute peripheral vestibular lesions, there is unidirectional horizontal and torsional nystagmus with quick phases beating away from the side of the lesion.

In the central lesions, bidirectional gaze-evoked nystagmus is seen, which could be vertical, typically downbeat, horizontal, or rotational, and importantly this nystagmus is not inhibited by fixation while the nystagmus due to peripheral lesions is inhibited by fixation.

Spontaneous nystagmus is observed with the patient looking straight ahead, while gaze-evoked nystagmus is noted with the patient fixating on targets 30° to the right, left, up, and down.

The Dix–Hallpike maneuver is done to elicit the positional and positioning nystagmus **(Fig. 4)**.

The Dix–Hallpike Positioning Test

This test is carried out by the examiner standing behind the patient who is seated on a couch.

The examiner holds the head of the patient and gently turns it 45° to one side and brings the patient down from sitting to lying position with the neck extended about 20° downwards from the couch. In this position, the eyes are observed for the occurrence of nystagmus for about a minute. If there is no nystagmus, the patient is brought back to the sitting position. This procedure is repeated after waiting for about 30 seconds with the head now turned to the opposite side. The patient should keep his eyes open throughout this procedure and fix his eyes on the examiner's nose. A

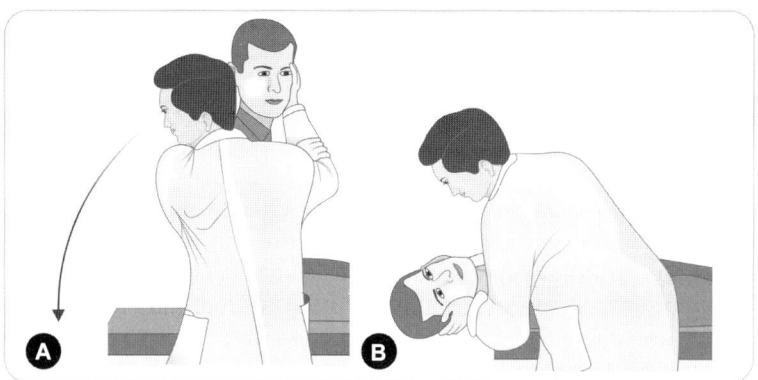

FIGS. 4A AND B: Dix–Hallpike test demonstration. Turn head to 45° (A) and bring the patient down from sitting to lying position with the neck extended about 20° downwards from the couch (B).

word of caution: Care should be taken in doing this test on a person with pain in the neck.

If a nystagmus occurs, its direction, duration, and importantly, the latency in its occurrence should be noted.

The Dix–Hallpike test is the gold standard test for eliciting positional nystagmus in persons with benign paroxysmal positional vertigo (BPPV) and is considered to have 50–80% sensitivity in its diagnosis. With posterior canal-induced BPPV, the nystagmus may appear after a short latent period, and hence the importance of observing for this latency in the up-beating and torsional nystagmus, which lasts for < 1 minute. For diagnosing lateral or horizontal canal BPPV, the supine roll or supine lateral head turns test is employed. This test is done when the Dix–Hallpike test is negative in a patient with BPPV.

The patient is asked to lie down in a supine position and the head is rotated 90° laterally to either side, one after the other, and the patient is instructed to keep the eyes open for examining the nystagmus. In lateral canal BPPV, the nystagmus is typically horizontal with no torsional component and there are two types of horizontal nystagmus which could be seen. The fast phase could beat toward the ground when it is called geotropic, or away from the ground when it is called apogeotropic, depending on the presence of otoconial debris within the lateral semicircular canal.

The otoconial debris gets dislodged from within the utricle and migrates into one of the semicircular canals during changes in head position. They float freely in the duct of the canal, resulting in abnormal endolymphatic flow within the affected canal (canalithiasis), or get adhered to the cupula of the canal (cupulolithiasis).

Head Impulse Test, Nystagmus, and Test of Skew (HINTS)

This battery of three tests has proved useful in the evaluation of AVS to detect brainstem and cerebellar strokes with greater sensitivity than even neuroimaging, according to Kattah et al.

Test of Skew

Skew deviation refers to a misalignment of the ocular axis in the vertical plane due to an imbalance in the firing of the vestibular neurons from the right and left. Skew deviation is detected by doing the alternate cover test. First, one eye is covered, and next the cover is shifted to the other eye. Refixation saccade is looked for in the uncovered eye. This test is done alternately **(Fig. 5)**.

The presence of skew deviation is strongly indicative of brainstem lesion.
A stroke can be identified by the presence of any one of these three signs:
1. Normal HIT
2. Horizontal nystagmus which changes direction according to the side of gaze
3. Presence of skew deviation

The mnemonic INFARCT would be useful in remembering these signs (*i*mpulse *n*ormal, *f*ast *p*hase *a*lternating, and *r*efixation on *c*over *t*est).

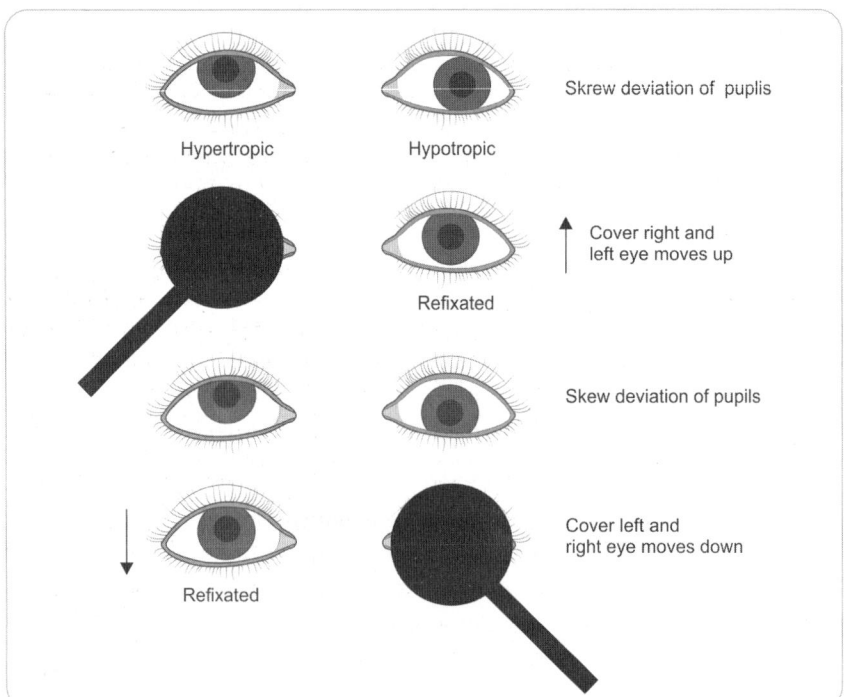

FIG. 5: Cover test for skew deviation.

HINTS Plus

The bedside hearing test was added to HINTS as the HINTS plus examination, to detect hearing loss due to cochlear or brainstem ischemia, and to increase the diagnostic accuracy in AVS and not miss a labyrinthine infarction.

Caloric Test

It is a fairly simple qualitative bedside test to assess the integrity of the lateral semicircular canals only and not the rest of the vestibular system. It is discussed further while dealing with investigations **(Table 1)**.

Other Bedside Clinical Examinations to Assess the Vestibular System (Flowchart 1)

Eye Movements Examination

This includes assessing the range of eye movements, looking out for the presence of gaze paralysis or internuclear ophthalmoplegia, and oculomotor paralysis.

TABLE 1: Differences between peripheral and central vertigo.

Characteristic	Peripheral	Central
Onset	Sudden	Gradual or sudden
Intensity	Severe initially, often decreasing over time	Mild in most but can be severe in stroke, and multiple sclerosis
Duration	Intermittent episodes lasting seconds to less than a minute in BPPV; continuous and lasting hours to days in vestibular neuritis	Usually weeks, or months (continuous) but can be seconds or minutes with vascular causes, such as posterior circulation TIA
Direction of nystagmus	Usually torsional and upbeat (fast phase beating toward forehead) in classic posterior canal BPPV; horizontal in horizontal canal BPPV; horizontal-torsional in vestibular neuritis/labyrinthitis	Purely vertical, spontaneous and purely torsional, direction-changing on lateral gaze, down beating (fast phase beats toward the nose)
Effect of head position	Induces vertigo (BPPV); worsens vertigo (vestibular neuritis)	Usually little change but can worsen with a head position change
Associated neurologic findings	None	Usually present
Associated auditory findings	May be present, including tinnitus (Ménière's disease) and hearing loss (labyrinthitis)	Rarely present

(BPPV: benign paroxysmal positional vertigo; TIA: transient ischemic attack)

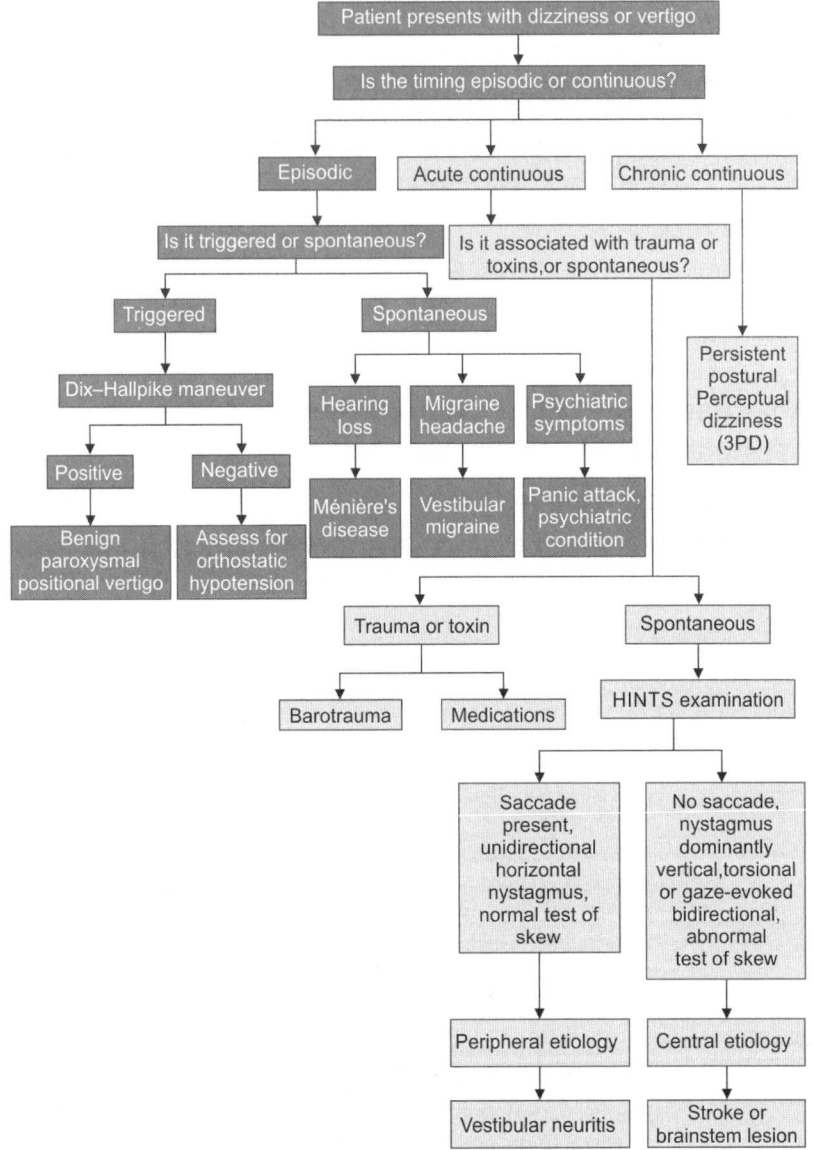

FLOWCHART 1: Algorithm of evaluation of dizziness.
(HINTS: head impulse, nystagmus, test for skew)

The assessment of eye movements would include looking at the saccadic, pursuit, and vergence movements. Abnormalities in these movements would indicate a central disorder. Saccadic movements are checked by asking the patient to look back and forth approximately 30° to each side or look at the ears of the examiner on either side horizontally, and also look up and down vertically. The latency, velocity, and accuracy of these movements are looked for. Delayed and slow saccades are seen in basal ganglia degenerative disorders, and inaccurate saccades, either falling short or over shooting are seen in cerebellar disorders.

Past-pointing Test

The patient, seated in front of the examiner should be asked to point at the examiner's extended index finger with his index finger extended but not touching it. Another test for past pointing is to ask the patient to raise his hands with the index finger pointing up and then bring down the hands to exactly touch the examiner's fingertips in front of him. This test is repeated several times with eyes closed and consistent deviation to one side is considered past-pointing and is indicative of cerebellar dysfunction.

Romberg Test

The patient is asked to stand with feet together and remain still with eyes closed. The test is considered positive if the patient loses balance, indicating either a proprioceptive sensory abnormality or a vestibular system dysfunction. A sharpened Romberg test could also be done by asking the patient to carry out the same maneuver with one foot placed in front of the other in tandem.

Tandem Walking Test

The patient is asked to walk in a straight line, placing one foot in front of the other, and this is a test of cerebellar function. Vision would compensate in chronic proprioceptive or vestibular dysfunction, and hence it is assessed better with eyes closed **(Table 2)**.

INVESTIGATIONS

The number of investigations available to assess vertigo and the balancing system, which is quite complex, is expanding, with more hi-tech gadgetry becoming available, though at an exorbitant cost. Hence, it becomes imperative for the physician to know the indications and the limitations of these multiple investigations, which would be of help in effectively managing the patient. These investigations can be categorized into those that indicate structural abnormalities and those that help assess the site of the lesion, the extent of the functional deficit, and the probable etiology.

Imaging Studies

CT scan and MRI are the imaging modalities and MRI would be the choice to delineate structural abnormalities of the brainstem and cerebellum; and hence, it needs to be done in all patients suspected to have a central cause for the vertigo and also in patients with AVS.

Imaging studies are also indicated in those with chronic vestibular syndrome (CVS) to exclude central nervous system (CNS) lesions. Among the conditions causing EVS, patients with definite features of BPPV and

TABLE 2: Advantages and limitations of the various clinical tests of the vestibular system.

Test	Description	Limitations
Dix–Hallpike maneuver	Test of individual posterior semicircular canal, for the diagnosis of posterior canal BPPV	• No reliable data on sensitivity and specificity • Nausea and vomiting can occur and should be avoided in cervical spine instability
Supine roll test	Test of individual horizontal semicircular canal, for diagnosis of horizontal canal BPPV	• Avoided in cervical spine instability • No comparative tests are available
Head impulse tests	Tests of high-velocity VOR. Most useful for subjects over the age of 60 years with > 60% unilateral vestibular weakness and no cervical limitations	• Not useful for younger adults or older adults with reduced cervical spine ranges • A negative response does not necessarily indicate normal vestibular function
Romberg test	Tests of standing balance	Not useful for patients with lower extremity peripheral neuropathy
Tandem walking	Test of walking balance	Problematic in patients with lower extremity peripheral neuropathy
Fukuda stepping test	• Subjects should stand upright with arms extended in front and close their eyes and walk in place. If the vestibular system is normal, they should not rotate to either side but may move forward • Rotation to the side indicates the impaired side	Not useful as a diagnostic test, or for rehabilitation screening

(BPPV: benign paroxysmal positional vertigo; VOR: vestibulo-ocular reflex)

vestibular migraine do not need imaging, as the diagnosis is based on clinical features. Imaging is required only for Ménière's disease in this group of disorders.

MRI is the imaging of choice for detecting strokes and structural abnormalities in the brainstem, cerebellum, and craniovertebral junction anomalies. A CT scan is useful for evaluating bony abnormalities of the temporal bone and the temporal canal.

Other tests are done to identify functional abnormalities in different areas of the balancing system. Many of these neurological investigations require sophisticated evoked potential recording systems and image processing modalities, apart from high technical skills, and a sound knowledge in interpreting the results by the investigator. It necessitates a test battery approach as balance needs normal functioning of several systems—the vestibular system, its central and peripheral pathways, the visual system, and normal cognition and psychology. No single test can comprehensively analyze the functioning of the vestibular and balance system and a combination of multiple tests would be required as each of these tests are like peep windows into the complex of the balance system. The tests and the structures evaluated are:

- Caloric testing for assessment of horizontal semicircular canals alone
- HIT, video HIT, electronystagmography (ENG) and videonystagmography (VNG) for all the semicircular canals and their connections
- Cervical vestibular-evoked myogenic potential (cVEMP) assesses the saccule, inferior vestibular nerve, and the structures involved in vestibulocollic reflex
- Ocular vestibular-evoked myogenic potential (oVEMP) evaluates utricle, superior vestibular nerve, and the structures involved in vestibulo-ocular reflex
- Subjective visual vertical with the bucket test is a test for multilevel localization
- Electrocochleography for assessing the integrity of the auditory hair cells
- Brainstem Evoked Response Audiometry (BERA) evaluates the retrocochlear auditory pathways

Caloric Test

This test is seldom done nowadays as it is cumbersome for both the patient and the examiner and has limitations.

An otoscopy should always be done before doing the caloric test to ensure that the tympanic membrane is intact and that there is no wax in the ear canal.

The head of the patient is elevated to 30° from the supine position to bring the lateral semicircular canal into a vertical orientation. Cold (around 30°C) or warm (around 42°C) water is used to irrigate the external canal which induces convection currents in the endolymph of the lateral semicircular canal.

The caloric test without ENG or VNG recording provides erroneous results and hence is best done with ENG or VNG recordings. It tests only the integrity of the lateral canal and the other two canals, the posterior and anterior, and the utricle and saccule are not tested by it.

No test in vestibulometry is a standalone test. A test battery is essential, as a normal finding in one test does not exclude a vestibular pathology. The test battery is quite expensive, and management directed information from it may be limited. Hence, the cost-benefit ratio should be considered before ordering such tests.

None of the tests can replace a thorough history and clinical examination. The tests only document the abnormality and have to be interpreted in conjunction with the history and clinical findings.

Vestibular Evoked Myogenic Potential Test (VEMP)

Of the abovementioned tests, the vestibular evoked myogenic potential (VEMP) test merits discussion as it is very often done. Its usefulness and limitation need to be understood. It is easy to do, does not require much time, is noninvasive, can be carried out with minimal training and is relatively inexpensive. However, its utility is not significant.

There are two components to the VEMP tests, the cervical and the ocular, denoted as cVEMP and oVEMP. These otolith-dependent reflexes are produced by stimulating the ears with air conducted sounds or skull vibrations and recorded from surface electrodes placed over the neck (cVEMPs) and eye muscles (oVEMPs). They are short latency, vestibular dependent reflexes.

The cVEMP tests the structural and functional integrity of the saccule and its afferent connections through the inferior vestibular nerve to the vestibular nucleus and from there through the median longitudinal fasciculus to the motor root of the accessory nerve to the sternocleidomastoid muscle.

This response is an electromyographic (EMG) recording of the sternocleidomastoid muscle brought about by the auditory stimulation of the saccule and represents an inhibitory vestibulo-collic reflex.

The 2 kHz normalized peak-to-peak cVEMP amplitude provides a 96% sensitivity and 100% specificity. The amplitude of the compound muscle action potential (CMAP) of the sternocleidomastoid muscle is compared on both sides and an asymmetry of > 35% indicates abnormality on the side with lower amplitude.

The oVEMP represents the active vestibulo-ocular reflex and the function of the contralateral utricle and superior vestibular nerve. VEMPs are used to determine the function of the otolithic organs namely the utricle and saccule of the inner ear. It forms only a small part of the vestibular function test battery and is not a standalone test. VEMPs are not of great help in general practice as it is normal in BPPV and migrainous vertigo, the two of the most common causes of episodic vertigo seen in practice.

■ DIFFERENTIAL DIAGNOSIS OF VERTIGO

Prior to the MRI era, great effort used to be taken to identify peripheral vertigo and differentiate it from central vertigo, as identification of central vertigo would necessitate invasive investigations. The availability of MRI now has made this differentiation less needed, though it is still good to know the clinical features that help differentiate central from peripheral vertigo, as it would help identify the conditions causing the vertigo.

PART 2

Disorders Causing Dizziness

DISORDERS CAUSING EPISODIC VESTIBULAR SYNDROME

Disorders causing dizziness could occur episodically or acutely or be persistent and chronic. These are disorders which occur intermittently as discrete episodes:
- Benign paroxysmal positional vertigo (BPPV)
- Migrainous vertigo or vestibular migraine
- Non migrainous benign recurrent vertigo
- Ménière's disease

BENIGN PAROXYSMAL POSITIONAL VERTIGO (BPPV)

Case Vignette

A 45-year-old lady comes with a history of experiencing a spinning sensation for 2 weeks following a blunt injury to her head on banging her head against a shelf in the kitchen. These episodes occur intermittently and last for less than a couple of minutes most often for a few seconds and occur associated with postural change like turning in bed, especially to the right side and lasts for a minute or two after which it spontaneously settles down. On occasions, she has similar symptoms on turning back to lie straight or in the left lateral position. She experiences rotation of surroundings with no associated nausea or vomiting. There is no history of tinnitus, fullness or pain in the ears, and she has not had similar episodes in the past. She is not a hypertensive but takes metformin for diabetes, which is under fairly good control. Neurologic, ear examination and hearing were normal. However, the Dix–Hallpike test was positive on the right.

Benign paroxysmal positional vertigo is probably the most common cause of vertigo. Most cases are idiopathic, and the next in frequency would be those following head trauma. Importantly, it could also occur concomitantly in association with other forms of vertigo or otological disease like Ménière's disease (MD) or vestibular neuronitis.

The pathophysiology could be either canalithiasis or cupulolithiasis. In canalithiasis, the otoconia are mobile and free-floating in the semicircular canals, and vertigo results from the force exerted by the otoconia within the canals. In cupulolithiasis, vertigo occurs due to densities caused by the adherent otoconia to the cupula of the crista ampullaris. BPPV is classified according to the semicircular canal involvement and posterior canal involvement is the most common one, being involved in 90–95% of cases of BPPV, followed by the lateral or horizontal canal in 5–15%.

The vertigo is of sudden onset, having a positional association, most often in a lateral position with the affected ear being down. The vertigo usually lasts for < 30 seconds of varying intensity. Obtaining a detailed history is critical as BPPV is a clinical diagnosis based on the symptom description, and some patients could also report an association of fogginess or clouding of brain functioning with BPPV.

The otological, head and neck, and neurologic examinations are invariably normal and the Dix–Hallpike test could confirm the diagnosis if it is positive.

Treatment

The treatment options include vestibular suppressants, canalith repositioning, vestibular exercise therapy, and in refractory cases, surgical management. Epley maneuver is the treatment of choice and is most often successful in repositioning the canalith in the posterior canal which is the common site of involvement. Lempert's supine roll maneuver is advised for canalith in the horizontal canal. These procedures reposition the canalith and relieve the symptom **(Figs. 1 and 2)**.

Vestibular exercises that help habituation and compensation are beneficial. Canalith repositioning and vestibular therapy are sufficient to alleviate in most instances. Surgical procedures of selective canal plugging or single nerve sectioning are reserved for the most refractory cases and are rarely required. BPPV can recur in about 15%.

Key Points

- BPPV is probably the most common cause of vertigo.
- The symptoms usually last for a few seconds.
- Canalith repositioning via Epley or Lempert maneuver is successful in giving relief of symptoms in most cases.
- Recurrence could occur in about 15%

■ MIGRAINOUS VERTIGO OR VESTIBULAR MIGRAINE

Case Vignette

A 34-year-old lady consults for giddiness since that morning. She experiences a spinning sensation in the head and feels comfortable only on

PART 2: Disorders Causing Dizziness

Illustration of the Epley maneuver and Lempert supine roll maneuver:

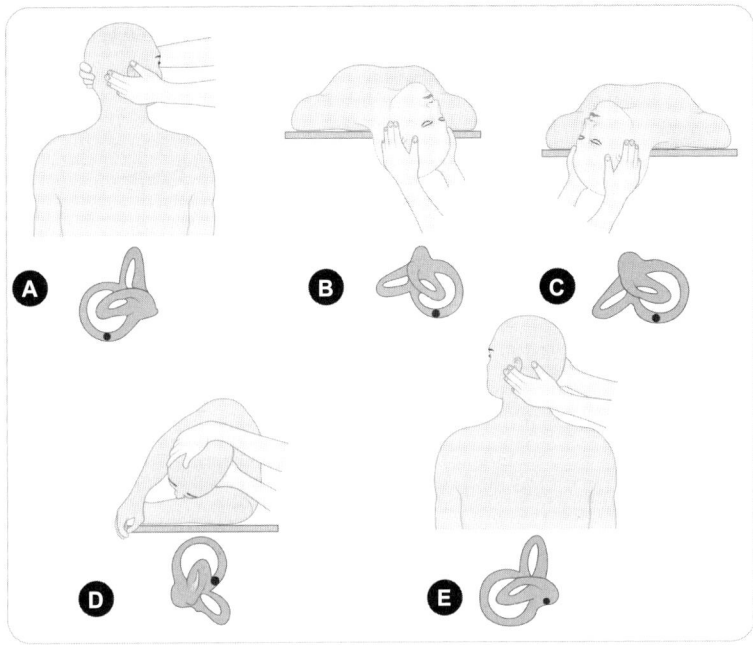

FIGS. 1A TO E: Epley maneuver for canalith in the posterior canal. (A) The patient is placed in the upright position with the head turned 45° toward the affected ear (the ear that was positive on the Dix–Hallpike testing). (B) The patient is rapidly laid back to the supine head-hanging 20° position, which is then maintained for 20–30 seconds. (C) Next, the head is turned 90° toward the other (unaffected) side and held for about 20 seconds. (D) Following this, the head is turned a further 90° (usually necessitating the patient's body to also move from the supine position to the lateral decubitus position) such that the patient's head is nearly in the facedown position. This is also held for 20–30 seconds. (E) The patient is then brought into the upright sitting position, completing the maneuver.

lying in a dark place. She has been experiencing such episodes for the past 2 years and the duration of such episodes would be from 2 hours to half a day and would settle down gradually with rest. Her concern is such episodes are happening more frequently of late and are associated with nausea and vomiting at times. She has been known to have migraine headaches since her teens and at present, the frequency of headaches has become less. When the headaches are severe, she would also have giddiness. However, at present, the dizziness is not associated with a headache on most occasions, though she does get mild-to-moderate headaches at times, along with the vertiginous sensation. There is no history of head trauma, and her medical history is unremarkable except for the above symptoms. Her clinical examination including her blood pressure is normal. The head impulse test (HIT) was normal. She had undergone an MRI evaluation of the brain earlier, which was normal.

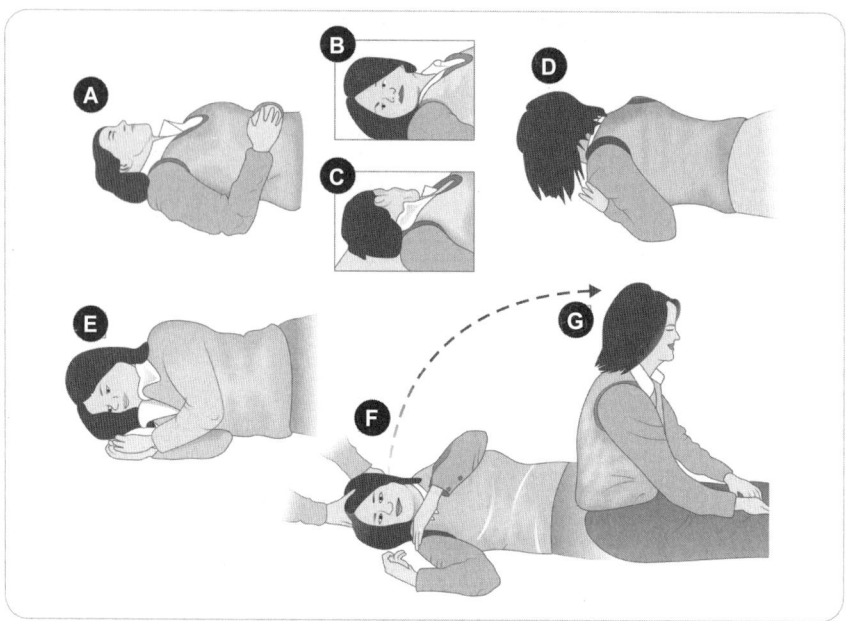

FIGS. 2A TO G: Lempert roll maneuver for canalith in the horizontal canal. (A) Start from the supine position. (B) Some recommend rolling to start on the involved side. (C) Roll his or her head (or full body) to the unaffected side. (D) Keep rolling in the same direction until his or her head is completely nose down or prone. Some recommend ending the maneuver here and returning to sit (270° roll) as anatomically the debris is repositioned. (E to G) As originally published, however, complete the final roll (full 360°), and return to sitting.

Migrainous vertigo is common, and in the opinion of the first author experience, is almost as common as BPPV. There is no gold standard diagnostic criteria for vestibular migraine, and it is one of the differential diagnosis in episodic vestibular syndrome (EVS). The diagnosis is essentially clinical, based on the description of the vertiginous episodes, and a normal clinical examination. Other differentials of EVS like BPPV, MD, can be excluded based on the description of symptoms, though a less-discussed entity of nonmigrainous recurrent benign vertigo, which shall be discussed later, needs to be considered as a differential.

The onset of symptoms is often gradual, though acute onset, is also described and the duration of symptoms ranges from 30 minutes to half a day, or at times the whole day. Headache need not always be an associated feature of the dizziness, though a considerable number of patients agree to experiencing giddiness when the headache becomes severe. However, in several patients, headache and vertigo occur at different times, and their respective frequencies also show shifting predominance. Rarely, patients do describe a cluster of vertiginous episodes occurring almost daily for a week to ten days at a stretch (personal experience), similar to cluster headache, but without a periodicity of recurrence.

The symptoms commonly described in association with vestibular migraine, are rotational and positional vertigo, often with intolerance to head and visual motion, and at times associated with motion sickness. Photo and phonophobias, and migraine triggers are also narrated by patients on specifically enquiring about them, and their presence strengthens the diagnosis. Migrainous vertigo is often described as experiencing a "boat-like" feel or a swaying motion.

The pathophysiology of vestibular migraine is thought to be the hyperexcitability of the vestibulo-trigeminal system, to a variety of stimuli such as bright lights, loud sounds, and self or environmental motion, during the episodes and at baseline.

There are no long-term studies as yet on migrainous vertigo or vestibular migraine and the natural history of this entity remains unchartered, though in the author's experience, it parallels that of migraine headaches without aura, and in women, the symptoms maximally occur during the childbearing years and then decrease in frequency and severity, after menopause.

Treatment

The mnemonic SEEDS outlines the lifestyle changes that help in the management of migraine and migrainous vertigo.
- *S*leep for at least 7 hours
- *E*xercise regularly
- *E*at at regular times as far as possible.
- *D*iary, making note of the frequency and duration of the attacks.
- *S*tress minimizing adaptations

Prophylactic agents used in the management of migrainous vertigo include:
- Tricyclic antidepressants (TCAs)
- Pizotifen
- Propranolol
- Topiramate
- Flunarizine
- Lamotrigine

Recently, the GEPANTS, calcitonin gene-related peptides (CGRPs), are used for the management of migraine headaches.

The abortive or rescue therapies for migrainous vertigo include vestibular suppressants, betahistines, cinnarizine, and triptans.

Key Points
- Migrainous vertigo or vestibular migraine is often described as a 'boat-like' feel or a swaying sensation.
- Photophobia and or phonophobia could be associated.

- This condition is much more common than Ménière's disease and could occur as frequently as BPPV.
- Treatment includes standard medications used to treat migraine.

Nonmigrainous Benign Recurrent Vertigo

This is a condition, that is not talked about or written about much, and yet is seen in practice, though not often. The symptoms are very much like those of migrainous vertigo and are characterized by recurrent episodes.

The vertiginous sensation lasts for a few hours, without tinnitus, earache or fullness, and on most occasions, without nausea or emesis. Some of these patients give a history of mild unsteadiness or a swaying feel during the period of giddiness. They neither have associated headaches nor give a history of migraine. They do not have triggers or photo or phonophobias, and these are the features that differentiate this condition from vestibular migraine.

Neurologic examination is normal, and an MRI brain reveals no abnormalities. Hence, they are considered benign, even though recurrent, and the nosology of this entity is far from clear at present. Treatment is empirical, and symptom relief with vestibular suppressants for the day of the symptom is adequate, as the recurrence of such episodes is usually infrequent. The natural course of the disorder is not known, as there is no proper study of this entity, but they do not develop new symptoms or deficits over time.

MÉNIÈRE'S DISEASE

Case Vignette

A male in his early sixties, presented with a history of vertigo of 4 days duration. The vertigo became severe with a change of position, disabling him in his normal activities because of a reeling sensation and a fear of falling and was associated with vomiting, though not on all occasions.

He has been having such episodes of vertigo, of varying severity over the past 15 years, but occurring infrequently. The frequency of these episodes would vary, with episodes occurring at intervals ranging from 3 months to 2 years and were invariably associated with tinnitus of varying severity and duration, before, and during the episodes of vertigo. He also agreed to be having a hearing deficit on the side of the tinnitus but was not sure about its progression.

Magnetic resonance imaging of the brain had been done twice in the past and was normal on both occasions. He used to receive vestibular suppressants during periods of vertigo from his physician.

Ménière's disease, also known as idiopathic endolymphatic hydrops, is not as uncommon as was thought to be earlier and is the third most common cause of EVS, after BPPV and vestibular migraine. It is a disease process involving the inner ear with a finding of fluid imbalance there (hydrops). The clinical significance of hydrops has, however, become controversial as recent studies have shown that hydrops alone may not be sufficient to cause the symptoms associated with MD.

The exact etiology is unknown, and it is believed to be multifactorial, with allergic, immunologic, autoimmune, and viral etiologic associations being hypothesized.

It typically presents as a unilateral disease, though bilateral presentations are known to occur. Over the course of the disease, unilateral involvement could progress to become bilateral, in about a third of patients.

The peak prevalence is between 40 and 60 years, though it could occur in the third decade itself. Familial association has also been reported. Ménière's disease is characterized by a tetrad of symptoms:
- Intermittent episodic vertigo
- Fluctuating hearing loss
- Tinnitus (low tone)
- Aural fullness (pressure or fullness sensation in the affected ear)

Clinical Presentation

The diagnosis is largely based on the history given by the patient. They have horizontal axis spinning or a subjective sensation of motion, and examination during periods of acute episodes could reveal horizontal or rotatory nystagmus. The episodes usually last for minutes to hours and could be severe and serial, and be associated with nausea, vomiting, sweating and pallor (autonomic symptoms). These episodes of vertigo could be preceded by increased tinnitus and sensorineural hearing loss, which are classical to this disease and are known as Lermoyez attacks, though these are not necessarily a constant accompaniment.

Ménière's disease is a disease characterized by remissions and exacerbations of varying severity with long periods of quiescence between attacks. Known triggers are periods, psychosocial stress, and certain dietary consumption.

The hearing loss is for low frequency, and in the early course, it fluctuates like tinnitus and could show improvement as well. However, as the disease progresses, both tinnitus and hearing loss could become permanent.

Sudden falls without loss of consciousness can occur in patients with MD and these drop attacks are known as Tumarkin attacks and could occur in clusters, although rare.

Diagnosis

The patient being asymptomatic between such distressing episodes, which might even necessitate visits to the emergency department, and having no abnormal clinical findings, is a good clue to the diagnosis of MD.

The diagnostic evaluation when MD is suspected should include pure tone audiometry to confirm the low-frequency hearing loss, although the hearing might be normal between the episodes in the early phase.

The most sensitive test for MD is electrocochleography, which is an electrophysiologic study that measures summating potential and the nerve action potential, in which the nerve action potential should be larger. A ratio > 0.4 is indicative of a hydropic state.

If the hearing loss and vertigo, which are noted, are not characteristic of Ménière's disease, an MRI of the brain needs to be done to look for pathology in the internal auditory canal or cerebellopontine angle indicating an alternate diagnosis.

The natural history of Ménière's disease is spontaneous remission over the years, though patients do have permanent vestibular deficits and hearing decline.

Treatment

Vestibular suppressants, such as meclizine, and diazepam, help abate the acute attacks but are not advocated for long-term preventive therapy. Conservative therapy should be tried given the high rate of spontaneous remission. Restriction of salt intake and avoidance of chocolate and caffeine is advisable. Diuretics have been shown to be beneficial. In those who fail on conservative measures, surgical management, including nonablative and ablative procedures, is advocated.

The nonablative procedures include endolymphatic sac decompression or intratympanic steroid instillation. Endolymphatic sac decompression has been shown to exhibit immediate success in about 75% of patients. Intratympanic steroid instillation is gaining ground in the treatment of acute episodes and in preventing the progression of the disease.

Ablative therapies include chemical ablation with intratympanic gentamicin injection, labyrinthectomy, or vestibular nerve sectioning.

Meniett Device

This device is a pressure equalization tube, allowing for pressure pulses to be delivered to the inner ear. The mechanism of action is not well understood but has been found to provide symptomatic relief with daily use.

Key Points

- Ménière's disease is associated with endolymphatic hydrops.
- Sodium restriction and diuretics are the first line of therapy.
- Steroid treatment appears promising.
- Associated neurologic signs, if present, warrant further investigation.

ACUTE VESTIBULAR SYNDROME

The disorders discussed hereunder occur with acute onset and has a monophasic course. Initial improvement occurs early within a week but thereafter occurs more gradually and can last for weeks. The causes could be infective, trauma, toxins, and idiopathic.

■ VESTIBULAR NEURITIS/VESTIBULAR NEURONITIS
Case Vignette
A 37-year-old female was admitted to the hospital because of persistent severe vertigo of 3 days duration with associated recurrent bouts of nausea and vomiting. Initial treatment in the emergency ward was of no avail and the symptoms persisted necessitating admission. She was conscious and did not have tinnitus, hearing loss, headache or photo and phonophobias. There was no past history of similar episodes, no head trauma, diabetes mellitus or hypertension. She had an upper respiratory tract infection a week earlier for which she had treatment.

She was a little obese and her blood pressure was normal. Neurologic examination showed nystagmus, which was horizontal with fast phase beating to the right. The rest of the examination was normal with no cranial nerve involvement or ataxia. Her hearing was normal on testing. Her MRI of the brain done by the emergency room staff at the time of admission was normal.

The term vestibular neuronitis was first coined by Dix–Hallpike in 1952. It is also known as idiopathic acute vestibular dysfunction, vestibular neuritis, and less commonly vestibular ganglionitis.

The etiology is not well understood. Infectious etiology has long been proposed and association with upper respiratory tract infections has been identified. Viral agents have been postulated and several studies have identified latent herpes simplex virus 1 as an associated factor.

Vestibular neuronitis can occur at any age, though the peak prevalence is noted between 30 and 50 years of age.

Clinical Presentation
The diagnosis of vestibular neuronitis is largely based on the history and clinical presentation, and it is an acute vestibular syndrome (AVS) presentation.
The characteristic features are:
- Vertigo
- Nausea and emesis
- Normal or unchanged hearing
- No additional neurologic findings

The onset of vertigo is most often sudden, and in the acute phase, it is quite severe, lasting for several hours to days, and becomes worse with movement, to the extent, that the patient is scared to move. Hearing loss is not associated, and this feature differentiates vestibular neuritis from labyrinthitis. Loss of consciousness, weakness, sensory symptoms or headaches are not features of vestibular neuritis and if present, should alert the physician to other etiologies and prompt investigations toward a brainstem or a posterior fossa pathology. During the later phase of neuronitis, the vertiginous symptoms abate, though the patient could experience disequilibrium, imbalance, or unsteadiness, which may last even for several weeks.

During the acute phase, the patient has horizontal or rotatory nystagmus which could be spontaneous or gaze induced. Head thrust test (HTT) if done, if the patient can tolerate the movement, would induce or enhance the nystagmus.

Natural History

Vestibular neuronitis is a self-limiting process and would resolve within hours or days of onset with residual disequilibrium, and instability resolving within weeks of the episode. Recurrence could occur though rare. However, these patients have an increased risk of having BPPV, and the pathophysiology of this occurrence is not clearly known. Loosening of the otoconia in the utricle following neuronitis or vascular injury has been postulated. Posterior canal BPPV, known as Lindsay–Hemenway syndrome, is commonly reported.

Treatment

Vestibular neuronitis is a self-limited disease and hence needs only supportive care.

Antiemetics are given to counter nausea and emesis, and if needed, intravenous fluids are administered for hydration. Vestibular suppressants are given during the acute phase as a short course to mitigate the severe vertigo and should not be continued for long for the residual disequilibrium, as it may compromise the central vestibular compensation. Antiviral therapy and corticosteroids have not shown beneficial effects on the outcome.

Most patients have some degree of permanent vestibular hypofunction following vestibular neuritis, and vestibular therapy is beneficial in facilitating compensation of unilateral vestibular hypofunction. Vestibular nerve sectioning might have to be resorted to in patients who do not improve with an extended course of vestibular rehabilitation and has been shown to have a good benefit.

Key Points

- Vestibular neuronitis or vestibular neuropathy is not associated with hearing loss
- The disorder is self-limited.
- Treatment is supportive.

LABYRINTHITIS

The presentation is that of acute onset of severe vertigo with sudden hearing loss.

Labyrinthitis is a disease process characterized by inflammation of the inner ear. The etiology is infective, either viral or bacterial. Autoimmune etiology related to Wegener's granulomatosis or polyarteritis nodosa has also been described. The viruses most often associated are cytomegalovirus (CMV) and measles. Bacterial labyrinthitis is due to the pathogens associated with otitis media or meningitis because of the anatomical contiguity. Changes happening within the labyrinth include cochleosaccular degeneration, endolymphatic hydrops, atrophy, fibrosis, fibro osteosarcoma proliferation in the sensory epithelia and support cells with secondary neuronal degeneration.

The above pathological changes give rise to the various clinical symptoms exhibited.

Clinical Presentation

The clinical features are similar to those of vestibular neuronitis, and the distinguishing feature is the hearing loss.

Tinnitus, aural fullness, otorrhea, otalgia, fever, and facial paresis could be the associated features, depending on the etiology. The hallmark features are sudden onset, nonepisodic vertigo, and hearing loss. During the acute phase, the vertigo could be severe, lasting for several hours to days and exacerbated by movements. Prolonged periods of dizziness, disequilibrium, or unsteadiness follow abatement of the continuous vertigo and might continue for weeks and even months.

Evaluation

The diagnosis is largely based on the clinical presentation. As with vestibular neuronitis, horizontal or rotatory nystagmus, spontaneous or gaze-induced, could be elicited at rest, or provoked on head thrust test (HTT). Weber examination with the tuning fork would lateralize to the contralateral ear. The presence of additional neurologic signs needs evaluation for an alternative diagnosis. Audiometric examination with pure tone audiometry varies with different etiologies of the labyrinthitis, and with viral labyrinthitis which is the most common one, high frequency sensory loss is seen in the involved ear. In suppurative labyrinthitis, a mixed loss with a conductive component can be identified and the hearing loss is associated with a higher degree of severe to profound sensorineural component. Labyrinthitis associated with meningitis could be associated with bilateral hearing loss. High resolution computed tomography (HRCT) of the temporal bones helps in the identification of the different aural causes of labyrinthitis especially mastoiditis. Some of the aural causes in the differential diagnosis include MD, ototoxic exposure, perilymphatic fistula, presbystasis, tumors in the internal auditory canal, cerebellopontine angle, and brainstem.

Ischemia in the anterior inferior cerebellar artery (AICA) territory should be an important consideration in patients with sudden onset of vertigo and hearing loss, and MRI needs to be done if cerebellar features are noted on examination.

Treatment

The treatment will vary depending on the etiology. Antibiotic therapy and operative treatment are indicated in suppurative labyrinthitis, and the operative interventions range from myringotomy to mastoidectomy in cases of complicated otomastoiditis or cholesteatoma. Cultures should be obtained to guide antibiotic therapy.

Supportive therapy is the mainstay of treatment of viral labyrinthitis and includes bed rest, adequate hydration, and antiemetics. Vestibular suppressants should be used for a short period during the acute phase to reduce the severity of vertigo and should not be continued indefinitely, lest they compromise central vestibular compensation. As with vestibular neuronitis, there is no definite evidence of improvement in outcome with antiviral therapy or corticosteroid use.

Vestibular therapy facilitates compensation in patients with long-term symptoms.

Key Points

- Labyrinthitis is associated with hearing loss which differentiates it from vestibular neuronitis.
- The etiology is most often viral, but bacterial and autoimmune etiology also should be considered.
- Treatment is based on the etiology.

▮ MAL DE DÉBARQUEMENT SYNDROME (MdDS)

This is a situational disorder characterized by symptoms occurring after disembarkation from a journey involving passive motion, within 48 hours.

The symptom is a nonspinning vertigo characterized by an oscillatory perception akin to rocking, bobbing, or swaying present continuously for most of the day and the symptom temporarily reduces during exposure to passive motion. With transient Mal de débarquement syndrome (MdDS), the symptoms resolve at or before 1 month, with the observation period extending up to the resolution.

In persistent MdDS, the symptoms last for more than a month.

Treatment

Medications rarely help in this disorder and include selective serotonin reuptake inhibitor (SSRI), serotonin and norepinephrine reuptake inhibitor

(SNRI), and TCAs. Benzodiazepines help as they make the patient care less about the symptoms. Vestibular rehabilitation also does not help much.

If there is no definite history of travel, then vestibular migraine has to be entertained.

SUPERIOR SEMICIRCULAR CANAL DEHISCENCE

Case Vignette

A 35-year-old lady presents with a history of vertigo following an injury to her chin by her son's forehead while playing basketball about a month ago. CT scan of the face done at that time did not reveal facial bone or mandibular fractures. The symptom reduced in intensity in a week, but thereafter, she experienced hearing her own voice to be loud and also echoing, and hearing her heartbeat and her footsteps in her right ear when she jogs. She experiences dizziness described as an arc-like movement of surroundings when she blows her nose, while vacuuming, during bowel movements, and whenever there is a loud noise in the environment. She does not have tinnitus, hearing loss, or vomiting.

The examination is unremarkable except for the Weber's tuning fork test lateralizing to the left ear.

An high resolution CT scan of the temporal bones showed dehiscence of the bone overlying the right superior semicircular canal.

Superior semicircular canal dehiscence (SSCD) is a relatively rare condition manifesting as an AVS.

Semicircular canal dehiscence represents an abnormal communication between the inner ear and the surrounding structure through a lack of osseous covering over the membranous labyrinth. This creates a third window in the inner ear, apart from the round and oval windows. Acute onset of vertigo with or without hearing loss occurs in dehiscence of any of the canals, though the superior canal dehiscence is the most common one.

Superior canal dehiscence is a process in which the superior bony covering separating the membranous labyrinth of the superior semicircular canal is defective and the membranous labyrinth is in contact with the overlying dura of the middle cranial fossa. The etiology of this dehiscence is believed to be most commonly related to the premature arrest in the development of the bone overlying the canal or congenital defects.

However, not all patients with evidence of dehiscence on radiology or post-mortem have a past history of symptoms consistent with the symptomatic disease.

Clinical Presentation

The characteristic presentation includes vertigo, oscillopsia, and hearing loss. Patients describe a sensation of vertical torsional movement as if the world is rotating on the face of a clock. The oscillopsia may be induced by loud sounds (Tullio phenomenon), changes in pressure in the ear canal transmitted to the middle ear (Hennebert's sign), or with the Valsalva maneuver. Normal environmental sounds could induce oscillopsia, disequilibrium, movement intolerances, and have been described along with other auditory complaints in SSCD.

Diagnostic Evaluation

Physical examination may reveal evoked eye movements of upward or torsional nystagmus on pneumatic otoscopy seen with superior semicircular dehiscence.

An HRCT scan of the temporal bone with 1 mm sections obtained in the vertical canal plane would identify the dehiscence in the superior canal.

Superior semicircular canal dehiscence mimics the presentation of perilymphatic fistula, and the other differentials include MD and BPPV.

Treatment

Treatment is oriented to the severity of symptoms. Avoidance of triggering stimuli would suffice for mild symptoms. In those with moderate symptoms, pressure equalization tube placement is advocated to prevent middle ear pressure during Valsalva. Operative repair is reserved for those with debilitating disease. Resurfacing and plugging of the canal are the two main techniques practiced and are effective in reducing the signs and symptoms.

Key Points

- Characteristic features of SSCD are vertigo, oscillopsia, and hearing loss.
- Tulio phenomenon may be present.
- The patient's tolerance of symptoms dictates the treatment needed.

CHRONIC VESTIBULAR SYNDROME

Chronic vestibular syndrome is characterized by persistent dizziness lasting for weeks and is associated with unsteadiness on walking, hearing impairment with unilateral vestibular loss or cerebellar degeneration.

Persistent Postural Perceptual Dizziness (3 PD)

- Persistent postural-perceptual dizziness (PPPD) (or 3PD in short)
- PPPD is a chronic functional vestibular disorder caused by a mismatch between visual and vestibular inputs and their processing mechanisms.
- It is not a structural or psychiatric condition.

Functional disorder is considered as one wherein the symptoms are incompatible with a known neurological or medical condition. The symptoms are genuine, but cannot be explained on the basis of a recognized 'organic' disease.

According to Professor Jon Stone, about 30–50% of outpatient visits in primary and secondary care are for functional disorders.
A positive diagnosis needs to be made based on:
- Symptom clusters, that are consistent and stereotyped.
- Presence of positive examination findings.
- It should not be a diagnosis of exclusion.

Persistent postural-perceptual dizziness usually follows an inciting event which is a balance challenging event.

These events could be BPPV, vestibular migraine, acute vestibular neuritis, a panic attack, or orthostatic hypotension (OH).

Persistent Postural-perceptual Dizziness is Characterized by
- *Persistent*: Characterized by chronic swaying for 3 months or more with symptoms of dizziness, unsteadiness or nonspinning vertigo
- *Postural*: Exacerbated with upright posture like standing or walking
- Perceptual as with active self-generated movement or passive movement like traveling in a car or elevator with exposure to moving traffic or complex visual stimuli like murals, phone visual materials, people in the mall.
- *Dizziness*: A false or distorted sensation of swaying, rocking, bobbing of oneself (internal nonspinning) or the surroundings (external nonspinning)

This condition reflects a maladaptive functional change, and its secondary effects include:
- Neck stiffness
- Gait disorder
- Fear of falling
- Agoraphobia
- Fatigue
- Dissociation

The most common age of occurrence is in the mid-forties and females outnumber the males. Clinical examination is usually normal with normal eye and inner ear findings, though the problem might have started with an insult to the inner ear, years earlier. The MRI of the brain shows no abnormality.

Recovery follows neuro-otological, medical and psychological therapies.

The treatment involves a multidisciplinary approach with a clear diagnosis and a realistic explanation of the nature of the condition.
Lifestyle modification as per the mnemonic of SEEDS in the forms of:
- *S*leep
- *E*xercise
- *E*ating
- *D*ehydration
- *S*tress management

Treatment of the underlying triggers which includes the pharmacological treatment with SSRIs and SNRIs, with effects independent of that on mood and are the most suited medications.

Selective Serotonin Reuptake Inhibitors
- Sertraline: 25 mg
- Escitalopram: 5 mg
- Fluoxetine: 10 mg

Serotonin and Norepinephrine Reuptake Inhibitor
- Venlafaxine: 37.5 mg
- Duloxetine: 20–30 mg (Staab 2020)

Psychological therapy with cognitive behavioral therapy (CBT) helps to reduce the threat response and improve the maladaptive coping mechanism.

Physical therapy improves balance, works on habituation, and reinforces the intactness of balance.

The emerging therapy for PPPD is vagal nerve stimulation (VNS) which results in an improvement in quality of life and depression scores, with a reduction in severity and exacerbations, of the vertiginous episodes with a decrease in anxiety, and a reduction of the postural sway.

The mechanism of action of VNS is not known, though a decrease in autonomic overactivation has been postulated. With treatment, there is a functional improvement in 70-80% of patients, though they may not achieve full restoration (Staab 2017). Without treatment, there is rarely a spontaneous improvement, and more often the situation worsens, with an increase in risk of anxiety, depression, and functional decline.

Key Points
- PPPD (3PD) is common, treatable, and is not a diagnosis of exclusion.
- Treatment often requires a multidisciplinary approach including education, vestibular therapy, selective medications, and treatment of mood disorder.
- Multiple vestibular disorders can coexist and potentiate each other, e.g., recurrent episodes of vestibular migraine can transform to 3PD.

▌VESTIBULAR PAROXYSMIA

Vestibular paroxysmia is a treatable neurovascular cross compression syndrome, due to arteries in the cerebellopontine angle causing pressure-induced dysfunction of the eighth cranial nerve.

The symptoms are recurrent, spontaneous, and short lasting, episodes of spinning or nonspinning vertigo, which last for less than a minute and occur with or without ear symptoms of tinnitus and hypo or hyperacusis. It can occur as a series of up to 30 attacks or more in a day.

The attacks may be triggered by particular head positions or hyperventilation and change of head position.

No central vestibular, oculomotor disorders or brainstem signs are present. The symptoms are usually triggered by direct pulsatile compression with ephaptic discharges and less often by conduction blocks, similar to trigeminal neuralgia.

Magnetic resonance imaging reveals the neurovascular compression of the eighth nerve in > 95% of cases, with a loop of the anterior inferior cerebellar artery, most often being involved. The posterior inferior cerebellar artery or the vertebral artery are much less often involved.

Most often, with there being a structural abnormality, signs of unilateral vestibular hypofunction could be elicited by head impulse test (HIT), head shaking nystagmus test, and caloric testing.

This condition is biphasic, with a peak in childhood, due to vertebrobasilar vascular anomalies, and later in the fifth and sixth decades, due to increasing atherosclerosis and vascular elongated ectasia of the blood vessel. Men are affected twice as often as women.

Treatment

The frequency of episodes can be reduced by antiseizure medications (ASMs) carbamazepine, oxcarbazepine, lamotrigine, and others.

Surgical treatment is reserved for medically intractable cases, when microvascular decompression is done, or in the rare instance of nonvascular compression by space occupying lesions, by resection of the lesion.

In children, the condition may resolve spontaneously since brain vascular and bony structures grow at different speeds.

Key Points

- Vestibular paroxysmia is an episodic vestibular disorder.
- Diagnosis is based on the patient's history of the symptoms, frequency and duration of the attacks.
- It is presumed to be due to compression of the eighth cranial nerve.
- ASMs ameliorate the attacks.

■ VESTIBULOGENIC SEIZURE OR EPILEPTIC VERTIGO

Epileptic vertigo is a form of partial seizures due to epileptic activity in the cortical region of the brain representing the vestibular system which is localized in the superior lip of the intra-parietal sulcus, the posterior portion of the temporal lobe, and the temporoparietal border zone.

Vestibulogenic seizures are characterized by brief spells of a 'spin' like sensation lasting a few seconds. Tinnitus, nausea, and nystagmus might occur. Contralateral paresthesia, olfactory, or gustatory symptoms may also occasionally occur, and loss of consciousness and generalized seizures could happen due to the spread of epileptic discharges to adjacent cortical areas.

Though vertigo as a manifestation of epilepsy was recognized by Hughlings Jackson in the 19th century itself, the concept found favor only recently (Saad 2011).

Diagnosis

The clinical description of the episode, given by the patient and or an eyewitness, is important for the diagnosis. The differentials include the other conditions that cause episodic vertigo, especially BPPV and vestibular paroxysms which are brief episodes, mimicking a seizure.

Electroencephalography (EEG) and MRI of the brain might help confirm the diagnosis and identify the seizure focus.

Vertiginous seizures respond well to ASMs used for treating partial seizures, carbamazepine, oxcarbazepine, and lacosamide.

Key Points

- Vertiginous epilepsy is a form of partial seizures arising from the vestibular cortical areas of the brain.
- Epileptic vertigo manifests as 'brief spins' lasting a few seconds.
- Vertiginous seizures respond well to ASMs, but at the same time, one must be aware that these medications themselves can cause dizziness.

■ DRUG-RELATED DIZZINESS

Drugs are not an uncommon cause of dizziness and are underdiagnosed. Kroenke and colleagues (2000) in their review, mention medication-related causes of dizziness upto 16%.

Drug-related dizziness is not easy to diagnose, especially in the elderly, as it may masquerade as an age-related symptom. There are a number of drugs and toxins that could cause dizziness or vertigo simulating peripheral and central vertigo.

A number of drugs could cause orthostatic hypotension (OH) which could cause dizziness, though not a true vertigo (pseudo vertigo). These include diuretics, alpha-adrenergic, calcium channel and beta blockers, amiodarone, and TCAs. Vasodilators, levodopa, dopamine agonists, and oral hypoglycemic agents can also cause dizziness.

Ototoxic medications can cause vertigo, and these are aminoglycoside antimicrobials, quinine, diuretics, antimitotic medications, and nonsteroidal anti-inflammatory agents.

A number of medications which have a depressant effect on the central nervous system, like anti-seizure medicines, neuroleptics, TCAs, benzodiazepines and opioids, can cause central vertigo and be associated with cerebellar ataxia, dysarthria, and nystagmus.

Treatment

Postural drop in blood pressure must be checked in patients who are on antihypertensives and vasodilators and complain of dizziness (pseudo vertigo). The blood pressure (BP) check is done immediately on standing and also after 3 minutes to look out for delayed orthostatic hypotension (DOH). Serum levels of antiseizure medicines would help confirm the medication's toxicity in those who are taking antiseizure medications.

The prognosis of drug-induced vestibular toxicity is variable, and it may even take several years for a normal functional recovery depending on the duration of exposure.

Vestibular rehabilitation and vestibular therapy, such as strengthening and stretching exercises, help. Recovery exercises to augment vestibular compensation, balance, and gait training exercises, enhance functional recovery.

Key Points

- Drugs and toxins cause dizziness quite often and are underdiagnosed.
- Recognition of pseudo vertigo, by drugs causing OH, and differentiating them from true vertigo, caused by other drugs, aids in better management.
- Vestibular rehabilitation and vestibular exercises enhance functional therapy.

ORTHOSTATIC DIZZINESS AND OTHER CAUSES OF DIZZINESS

Hemodynamic Orthostatic Dizziness or Vertigo

The diagnostic criteria include:
- Five or more episodes of dizziness, unsteadiness, or vertigo triggered by arising (i.e., change of body posture from lying to sitting or standing) or present during upright position which subsides on sitting or lying down.
- OH, postural orthostatic tachycardia syndrome (POTS) or syncope are documented on standing or during head-up tilt test.
- Not documented as another disease or disorder

POSTURAL ORTHOSTATIC TACHYCARDIA SYNDROME

Case Vignette

A lady in her late twenties sought consultation for episodes of headaches and dizziness occurring together and independently for about 2 years' duration. She had undergone functional endoscopic sinus surgery (FESS) for her symptoms of headaches, but the episodes of headaches continued. Dizziness was said to be associated with palpitations and fear, and at times, was the predominant manifestations making her take emergency consults. Repeated taking of history at reviews revealed that quite often the headache was of a coat hanger distribution and was associated with dizziness and palpitations when she stands up erect.

Over time, it became established that she had an increased heart rate of > 120 beats/min during such episodes and there was a variability in heart rate with an increase of > 30 beats/min when examined during such times. However, her BP showed no fluctuations and remained normal.

She was put on propranolol with a diagnosis of POTS and was also reassured, explaining the nature of her problem. The episodes of headaches and dizziness became less and after getting convinced of the nature of her illness, the panic also was considerably reduced. She reduced and discontinued the medication when she was well after 3 months of medication, though she continued to have symptoms infrequently. During these times, she would take propranolol on her own for 10–15 days as necessary. Over a 6-year follow-up, she is doing well with occasional episodes of symptoms related to posture.

Postural orthostatic tachycardia syndrome can be:
- Primary as idiopathic, partial dysautonomic, and hypoadrenergic
- Secondary due to Ehlers–Danlos, immune-related, autonomic neuropathy, and hypovolemic state
- More often seen in females, and in the age range of 14–50 years.

Diagnosis

It is established by documenting an increase in heart rate of 30 beats or more per minute or 40 beats if < 18 years of age within 10 minutes of standing or being upright on a tilt table and with no drop in BP.

Several theories have been postulated though none has been established as the mechanism, and there is not enough data on the treatment either.

Treatment

Often treated with fluids, increased intake of sodium, and exercise. The medications include fludrocortisone 0.1–0.2 mg, beta blockers, pyridostigmine 60 mg thrice daily, and Ivabradine 2.5–7.5 mg twice daily.

Outcome

About one-third of patients improve and do not have POTS at 12 months

Delayed Orthostatic Hypotension

Quite a number of elderly patients have DOH which goes unrecognized. They have dizziness which is at times associated with falls also.

By definition, there should be a drop of 20 mm Hg. or more, of systolic BP, or a drop of 10 mm Hg or more of diastolic BP occurring after 3 minutes of standing up or being upright on tilt table testing.

Key Points

- DOH might be the reason for dizziness with or without syncope, in middle-aged or elderly people.
- Over a period of 10 years, more than half of those with delayed OH go on to develop OH, and parasympathetic autonomic system abnormalities.
- About 25% develop neurodegenerative diseases, most commonly alpha synucleinopathies – Parkinson's disease, dementia with Lewy bodies, multisystem atrophy
- The 10-year mortality is greater in delayed OH than in age-matched controls.

Dizziness and Hypertension

High BP could be associated with dizziness. Vertigo occurs in up to 20% of hypertensive patients and is unrelated to elevated BP but could be due to associated BPPV.

Synopsis

Dizziness is a symptom confronting the physician very often. There are as many causes of dizziness as there are descriptions, encompassed in that all-inclusive term. A detailed and accurate history is pivotal to approaching this complex symptom and formulating appropriate treatment for the cause of the symptom, rather than just providing symptom relief.

Vertigo is the most common form of dizziness met within neurology and neuro-otological practice and has to be sifted out of the many disorders enumerated earlier.

The diagnosis of the conditions causing vertigo, is most often clinical, based on the history and clinical examination, and seldom requires extensive investigations.

Triaging the types of dizziness and classifying syndromically, based on the history of evolution of the symptom into acute, episodic, and chronic vestibular syndromes, helps narrow down the differential diagnosis to a great extent and provides guidance for appropriate treatment.

SUGGESTED READINGS

1. Bisdorff A, Von Brevern M, Lempert T, Newton-Toker DE. Classification of vestibular symptoms: towards an international classification of vestibular disorders. J Vestib Res. 2009;19:1-13.
2. Staab JP. The influence of anxiety on ocular motor control and gaze. Curr Opin Neurol. 2014;27:118-24.

3. Bhattacharyya N, Baugh RF, Orvidas L, Barrs D, Bronston LJ, Cass S, et al. Clinical Practice guideline: benign paroxysmal positional vertigo. Otolaryngol Head Neck Surg. 2008;139(5 suppl 4):S47-81.
4. Kim JS, Zee DS. Clinical Practice. Benign paroxysmal positional vertigo. N Engl J Med. 2014;370:1138-47.
5. Alexander TH, Harris JP. Current epidemiology of Menier's disease. Otolaryngol Clin North Am. 2010;43:965-70.
6. Strupp M, Brandt T. Vestibular Neuritis. Semin Neurol. 2009;29:509-19.
7. Strupp M, Brandt T. Peripheral Vestibular disorders. Curropin Neurol. 2013;26:81-9.
8. Neuhauser H, Lempert T. Vestibular Migraine. Neurol Clin. 2009;27:379-91.
9. Kattah JC, Talkad AV, Wang DZ, Hsieh Y-H, Newman-Toker DE. HINTS to diagnose stroke in the acute vestibular syndrome: three-step bedside oculomotor examination more sensitive than early MRI diffusion-weighted imaging. Stroke. 2009;40(11):3504-10.

Index

B
BPPV 17

C
Caloric test 15
Canalithiasis 18
CGRP 21
Cupulolithiasis 18

D
Dix Hallpike 8
Disequilibrium 2

E
Epley maneuver 19

G
GEPANTS 21

H
Hennebert's sign 6
HINTS 10
HIT, HTT 6
Hydrops 23

L
Labyrinthitis 26
Lempert maneuver 19
Lermoyez attacks 23

M
Mal De Debarquement Syndrome 28
Ménière's disease 22
Meniett device 24

N
Nystagmus 8

O
Orthostatic hypotension 34

P
POTS 35
PPPD 30
Presyncope 2

S
SEEDS 21
Skew 10
SNRI 32
SSRI 32

T
Tullio phenomenon 30
Tumarkin attacks 23

V
VEMP 16
Vertigo 2
Vestibular Neuritis 25
Vestibular paroxysmia 32

INDEX